LOSING WEIGHT: A HERO'S JOURNEY

Dr. Denis Boucher, Ph.D.

ISBN 978-2-9813271-8-5 (Print)
ISBN 978-2-9813271-9-2 (EPub)

Edited by Allan Ross (AllanRoss.com)
Cover page and publishing: Ublo.ca

WARNING

The purpose of this publication is to guide you in your weight loss efforts. Application of the information provided in this publication in no way guarantees results. The contents of this publication are provided for information purposes only and do not constitute a professional opinion on any subject whatsoever. This publication cannot, in any manner, be deemed a substitute for the advice of a qualified physician, health care professional, nutritionist or physical fitness professional. Always seek the advice of a qualified health care professional regarding any questions you may have concerning your medical condition and your state of health before undertaking any weight loss or fitness program as presented in this publication. Any issues regarding your health require monitoring by a health professional. Neither your acquisition nor use of this publication establishes a physician-patient relationship, or any other therapeutic relationship, between you and the author. Furthermore, neither the author nor any other person associated with this publication shall be liable for any injury, loss or damages to any person acting, or refraining from acting, directly or indirectly on any information contained in this publication. Lastly, the application of techniques, ideas and suggestions presented in this publication is to be carried out solely at the discretion and risk of the reader.

Without limiting the generality of the foregoing, if you have any muscle or joint problems, health problems, cardiovascular or pulmonary disorders, health risk factors such as tobacco use, hypertension, diabetes, high cholesterol, stress, or if you experience fatigue or shortness of breath, it is important to obtain your physician's authorization before starting any fitness program.

The examples of discussions and conversations with clients in this publication are general summaries intended to preserve client anonymity and confidentiality of information.

TABLE OF CONTENTS

PART 1
THE TRUE MEANING OF THE EXPRESSION "LOSING WEIGHT"

01
A HISTORY OF WEIGHT LOSS

My formative experiences as a weight loss coach go back many years. At the time, I had been contracted by a pharmaceutical company that had recently launched a weight loss medication to provide guidance to patients who were using this medication.

From that moment, I began to realize that the "world" of weight loss had something odd, complex and fascinating about it.

I remember one of my first clients. He was 170 cm (5.58 ft) tall and when I measured his waist line, I was amazed to see that the measuring tape read a whopping 157 cm (5.15 ft). My conclusion was "Wow! I've never seen this before. This fellow is almost as round as he is tall!" He must have noticed that I was totally taken aback for him to say: "So you're the one who'll be performing miracles for me," to which I replied, "I don't see how I can lose weight for you, sir."

There's also this other client who came into my office beaming with joy to tell me: "This is really great! This means that with this medication, I'll be able to eat even more!"

And then there was this couple. When I explained to them that they would no longer be able to go through a large bag of chips every night, the woman burst into tears and said: "I hope it won't be like that for the rest of our lives?"

Although deep down I already knew it, this is the moment where I really "understood" the extent to which human behaviour plays a major role in weight gain. I also realized that, in many cases, nothing more can be done. No one can help people who don't want to help themselves.

This was also the time when I was finishing up my doctoral studies in experimental medicine. Scientific knowledge about weight loss was primarily based on the mathematical model (more on this subject later) and the quasi-irrational fear of consuming lipids. That's right, even weight loss "science" was limited to: consuming as few calories as possible, reducing your fat intake as much as possible and spending as many calories as you can through exercise. There was something of a scientific consensus in this regard, but the problem was that few scientists realized that the people following these recommendations were simply unable to lose weight or, if they did, their success was merely temporary.

Also at that time, cardiologist Dean Ornish demonstrated the effectiveness of a vegetarian diet on the reduction of atherosclerotic plaques (plaques that build up and end up blocking arteries). Although effective, this was just a passing fad.

At the hospital where I was studying, I attended a conference by Michel Montignac, who had come to explain the tenants of his theory, which was highly popular at the time, to physicians and scientists. This was another approach that demonstrated its effectiveness, but also lost considerable significance over the years.

Thus, from my perspective, there were only broad theories, but nothing could explain the mechanisms by which a person stores or burns fat. We appeared to still be lacking a lot of knowledge.

My greatest joy was to have access to an exercise physiology lab, which allowed me to measure the metabolism (use of energy reserves) at rest and under effort. One of my first observations: each person's metabolism is specific to that person and reacts in its own way to the various demands from the person's environment. So then, how could a single weight loss theory have allowed a large number of people to lose weight whereas, at the metabolic level, every person is different and reacts differently to the various demands of their environment? In short, I observed, I asked questions, but I still wasn't getting any satisfactory answers.

One day, I sat down with my doctoral research director and told him: "We have one of the most sophisticated exercise physiology labs in the world, yet I have the feeling that we could do so much more; learn much more about how metabolism works at rest and under effort." In his own unique way, his answer helped me understand: "It's there to be used, so use it and learn."

I then began my first experiments. One of my strangest, yet supremely rewarding, experiments was to place the subjects on a treadmill, hook them up to an electrocardiograph machine, ask them to walk and then assess their physiological reactions in real time. So far, nothing special, right? But I added a little spice to the mix. Before the start of the experiment, I asked the subjects to identify situations they considered to be stressful. As they walked on the treadmill, I asked them to talk about these situations out loud so that I could record their "speech." The variety of reactions I observed was astounding! This was troubling to me, as I could lose myself faced with so many different psychological reactions, but it was fascinating because no two people reacted the same way. Each subject's metabolism tried to adapt in different ways to the environmental demands (in this case, a psychological stressor). I knew something very important was hidden here but, once again, I couldn't quite put my finger on it.

Once my doctoral studies were completed, I had already started my own business operating an exercise physiology lab from which I could analyze metabolism at rest and under effort. Over the years, long after the initial and most difficult years in business, my lab became more and more successful, and I was able to complete thousands of tests. Thousands of observations of how metabolism works at rest and during exercise.

So then, after countless tests and observations, I finally understood. The body (metabolism) manages its energy reserves in such manner as to respond, to the best of its abilities, to the demands of the environment, and its main task is to survive. I hadn't invented anything – I just finally understood, and especially "measured," what this really meant.

My data showed that there was a type of central ZONE where the body was able to adapt and two extreme zones where it deteriorated: sedentariness coupled with inadequate nutrition, and high-intensity training coupled with food deprivation. In the first case, the body stores fat because the energy reserves are hardly used and in the second case, the body stores fat to survive the physiological stress to which it is subjected.

I had finally found the answer I was looking for. But, was I right? That's when I started attending scientific conferences where the world's leading scientists in my field presented the findings of their research. What a thrill it was to realize that I wasn't the only one to understand metabolism through this angle!

So, I was right. The next step was to put these findings into practice. This led to the launch of my weight loss program based on an analysis of metabolism at rest and under effort.

From the start, my program generated excellent results for most of my clients. However, I was well aware of the fact that to improve my program, I had to understand what led some people to resist losing weight.

My weight loss-resistant clients pushed me to explore the reasons behind this problem. The first answer I found was fairly simple. Some people say they want to lose weight but don't act accordingly. That's when I realized what the term "losing weight" meant at a human level. In fact, I define losing weight as follows: reaching a healthy weight and maintaining it for the rest of one's life. This is a sizeable challenge, as losing weight isn't enough. It is essential that a person acquire and maintain new behaviours for the rest of his or her life. This is why I've never wanted to present my program as a kind of miracle approach that promises quick weight loss. I preferred working with reality right from the start: losing weight is a considerable challenge that few people have the courage to face. I therefore shaped my program accordingly.

The second answer to the problem of weight loss resistance was just as obvious, but not as easy to control. We live in a world that demands a lot from each and every one of us. We subject our bodies to intense demands to which it is biologically unable to respond over the long term. Stress, insomnia, long work hours, multiple health problems, modern nutrition, sedentariness, exhaustion from exercise, lifestyle habits, etc. represent a set of factors that affect metabolism to a degree that makes weight loss nearly impossible. The body tries to survive this intense psychological stress, and it needs to store fat to survive. Under these conditions, the body is only doing its job. Under these conditions, a person who wants to lose weight must do a little "housecleaning" in his or her own life. Is this always possible? Does the person want to actually undertake this "housecleaning?" There are no set answers to these questions.

From that point forward, losing weight to me touched upon human and metabolic dimensions that are closely related. Clients cannot be separated into different components; I had to consider them from a human perspective as a whole.

Oddly enough, I saw certain similarities between my approach to weight loss and other areas of life. For example, some of my friends wanted to succeed in business. Talking about it was easy, but getting it done was another story. And for those who decided to act on their intentions, to achieve positive results, they had to apply good strategies (behaviours) and repeat them day after day for the rest of their lives. But, it's easy to forget this when you don't use the right tools. Many people consider work volume to be a guarantee of success. But how many people become exhausted before they achieve satisfactory results? Too many. And, when difficulties arise, they have to have the necessary strength to call themselves into question and find the right path back to success. These problems reveal who we really are. Do we give up or do we push forward at this time? This is not a journey in which everyone can be successful.

I now know that "losing weight" is not simply a reflection of the drop in the numbers on the bathroom scale. Successful weight loss is a major challenge, as it touches upon the deepest aspects of being human.

To lose weight, my clients must become aware of this hard and implacable truth. Now, I will tell you what I teach my clients on a daily basis. As for the rest, you are the only person who can do what it takes to lose weight. The real question is: are you ready to do what it takes? To answer this question, I invite you on this epic journey. A journey that only heroes can undertake.

02
A FEW MOMENTS TO THINK BEFORE WE BEGIN

For most people, losing weight simply means lower numbers on the scale. The faster they can achieve this, the faster they can go back to their good old lifestyle habits and regain all the weight they lost, and then some.

If you stop for a moment to think about how absurd this is, you will realize that losing weight represents much more than the pounds you shed. Why? Because the real goal is to achieve a healthy weight and to maintain it for the rest of your life.

I can already hear you say: "Yes, Denis, that's the real goal of losing weight." Very well, then, here's another question: What are the implications of this goal? Carefully read the answer:

1. You have to follow a specific plan.
2. You have to invest time in the process.
3. You have to follow your plan for the rest of your life.
4. You have to change your lifestyle.
5. You have to realize that your excuses to justify overeating no longer work.

Achieving a healthy weight and maintaining it for the rest of your life is not an easy task, as you will have to acquire new behaviours and have the necessary courage to apply them day after day. In doing so, you will build a new lifestyle for yourself, which will enable you to achieve your goal.

The reality is that this goal (achieving a healthy weight and maintaining it for the rest of your life) is not something you can accomplish in just a few months. You will have to maintain your new lifestyle for the rest of your life. Reverse course for a few months and you will gain back all the weight you lost. Isn't this an unbearably unfair and ruthless reality? Sure it is, but it's the truth. So, all of the best excuses in the world to justify not doing what you have to do, such as: "we have to enjoy life from time to time," will never prevent you from gaining weight. You can try to make yourself feel better by telling yourself: "It's not that bad," but your body is totally oblivious to what you believe; all it's doing is managing its energy reserves (calories) as best it can. Abuse it and it will store fat, even if you firmly believe that things aren't all that bad.

Losing weight is a process, a journey for heroes. Heroes that accept all that is involved in "achieving a healthy weight and maintaining it for the rest of your life." Few people are truly prepared for this. At this point, be brutally honest with yourself and ask yourself whether YOU are truly ready for this.

I know, you are really motivated and your answer is "YES, Denis, I want to go ahead with this." Then welcome aboard. But wait, you think it's that easy. You will come across many obstacles: stagnant weight, temptation, your good old excuses, slacking off, the difficulties and stress of daily life, your emotions, lack of time, etc. You'll encounter many enemies on this journey. What will you do? Do you feel up to the challenge of facing all these situations?

I cannot overstate this fact: losing weight is for heroes. Not for people looking for a miracle approach to losing weight fast. Losing weight is for heroes, people with a long-term outlook determined to overcome the many difficulties they will come across. Losing weight is for heroes that don't get discouraged at the first hurdle, only to hop right back into their old lifestyle habits that brought on all that excess weight in the first place.

Losing weight is for heroes. Do you have what it takes? That is the real question.

03
YOUR BODY IS THE ONLY ONE YOU'LL HAVE IN THIS LIFETIME

Your body is the only one you'll have in this lifetime. It is through this body that you will express yourself and communicate with the people around you.

Losing weight essentially reflects a wish to appreciate your own body. While it is true that the main motivating factor for some people is their health, the reality is that most people want to have a body they are happy with. And, there's nothing wrong with that.

When extra weight or obesity jeopardizes your perception of your body, which no longer represents the person inside you and what you want to express through it, you know that the time has come to do something about it.

This notion bears repeating: I believe that being proud of your appearance is a good thing. All too often, however, this goal of having a body you're happy with makes you want to lose weight quickly, because you want to get rid of this feeling of dissatisfaction with your body as quickly as possible.

This, however, is not the real goal. The real goal behind losing weight is to **achieve a healthy weight and to maintain it for the rest of your life**.

I can hear you thinking: "But Denis, what's the difference? I simply want to lose weight!"

All right. But if your goal is to get rid of the dissatisfaction you feel about your body as quickly as possible, what are you going to do? You'll want to lose weight as quickly as possible. And what do people do when they want to lose weight quickly? They go on a crash diet and train to exhaustion. And what are the actual results of this? You already know the answer, as you've been through this many times. Once the weight is gone, it all comes back, and then some, in the weeks or months ahead. Under these circumstances, no one can claim success.

So, since the real goal is to **achieve a healthy weight and maintain it for the rest of your life**, this means that your vision of weight loss, your actions and your behaviours must change.

Instead of spending your whole life going from one diet to another and always falling back to square one, you have to find and maintain a life balance that will enable you to achieve a healthy weight and maintain it for the rest of your life.

To achieve this, you have to change your lifestyle. And that, folks, is for heroes.

04
THE EMERGENCY OF LOSING WEIGHT

All these ideas make sense to you, don't they? But there you are, standing in front of the mirror and... panic sets it. "No way, that's not me. How could I have gained so much weight? This makes no sense. I HAVE TO DO SOMETHING ABOUT THIS RIGHT AWAY!"

And the panic fogs up your brain. The situation becomes unacceptable to you and gives rise to this short-lived motivation – which appears in the form of an internal sense of emergency – that acts as a call to action.

And, these "ALARM BELLS" going off obviously require a radical solution.

Without thinking, you take the bull by the horns and go for the same old strategy as before: a radical diet and high-intensity training to burn off as many calories as quickly as possible.

And since you've read all about this new miracle diet that, in combination with a high-intensity exercise program that includes 92 daily training sessions of 12 seconds each (ok, I'm being a little facetious), that promises a 20-lb weight drop in half a day (I can't help myself...), you're all in. "Yes, I can feel it, I've got it now, it's going to work this time! I have to stay motivated, I'm going to make it! Yes, I'm sure about this. This is going to work for real!"

But, under the cover of this new miracle approach, you don't realize that this is the exact same strategy that led you to failure in your previous weight loss attempts. The same strategy that led you to failure your entire life, perhaps... This approach boils down to this: food deprivation and exhaustion through exercise. If failure was the result of each and every previous attempt using this type of strategy, why should it work this time? Should it work because you believe in it more than you did the last time? Come on, you know it won't work any better this time around.

Instead of once again charging headlong into a wall of deception, take the time to implement this all-new strategy that I am suggesting to you: life balance. No, nothing spectacular, no bells and whistles, but it's the only strategy that really works.

By taking the time to implement the plan that will enable you to achieve a healthy weight and maintain it for the rest of your life, you can no longer let panic serve as your guide. Instead of smashing into a wall of deception yet again, you can regain control of your life and your body.

But, this vision of life, of weight loss, is for heroes. Isn't it time for you to become the hero in your own life?

05
YOUR WORST ENEMY

"Ninety percent of weight loss happens between your two ears." This statement may appear exaggerated, but it simply expresses the fact that your thoughts, emotions and behaviours determine a major part of your success (once you have applied the right weight loss strategy).

To properly illustrate this concept, let's consider an example of the type of discussions I have with some of my clients throughout their weight loss process.

First month

— Congratulations! You lost 8 lb the first month. That's excellent!

— Yes, I'm really happy Denis. I followed the plan to the letter.

— All right, then. I'll give you a grade of 100%. You're off to a great start, and I strongly recommend that you continue with the plan as it stands for the next month.

Second month

— Congratulations once again! You lost 6 lb in the second month. Great work!

— Yeah, I guess so... I'm not sure. I didn't follow the plan to the letter this time. I had several business dinners and there was plenty of booze... You know how it is, Denis...

— Sure, I do, but tell me something. Did you *have* to drink that much alcohol?

— Um... no. But the thing is you don't really notice... They keep refilling your glass and that adds up to a lot of alcohol.

— Yes, I know, but were you required to drink? Did anybody force you to?

— No, it's just difficult in those types of situations. You understand, don't you Denis?

— But life is full of these types of situations full of temptations. Haven't you understood that to achieve your goal you had to develop better control of a situation and of your own self?

Third month

— Denis, I'm not very proud of myself; I know I've gained weight.

— You did indeed. Since our last meeting, you've gained 3.5 lb. What happened?

— You see, Denis, it's summer and I find it a lot harder. There are so many opportunities to drink and eat things I shouldn't.

— I know, but it's like that for everyone. But you, what do *you* really want?

— I don't want to be obese anymore. I really want to lose weight.

— Well then, if you really want to lose weight, even though it's summertime, simply go back to the original plan we put together. Do you think you can handle that?

— Sure, Denis. That's what I'll do, I promise.

Fourth month

— Denis, I'm really ashamed and disgusted with myself. I've lost control and I have to make up for it.

— Other than eat too much, what did you do?

— Well, since I'm eating more calories, I exercise a lot more to compensate...

— So, you try to compensate for one imbalance with another... Isn't that what you've done your whole life and doesn't that explain why you're obese today?

— But Denis, I thought I was doing the right thing.

— No, you didn't think you were doing the right thing, you just want to go back to your old habits and hope to somehow lose weight anyway.

— You're probably right.

— Don't you see? Losing weight is based on living a balanced life. Why don't you make a definitive choice today?

— What choice is that?

— If you want to drink and eat whatever you like, choose to stay obese... Who could hold that against you, since it will be your choice and you will stop lying to yourself?

— But Denis, that's not what I want.

— Well then, if you really want to lose weight, stop complaining, trying to find excuses and justifications and trying to manage one imbalance with another... Do what needs to be done: follow the original plan... If you recall, the one that worked right from the beginning.

I know what you're thinking: "Denis, you're ruthless. Aren't you ashamed to be speaking to your clients like that?" My answer to that is: No. The way I see it is, they pay me to tell them the truth. If the conclusion of this discussion left you feeling a little shaken up, could it be that it reflects behaviours that you don't want to see in yourself?

Your excuses, your belief in being able to go back to your old lifestyle habits without causing any damage, chastising yourself to relieve your conscience, and managing one imbalance with another... This is how you become your own worst enemy. And this enemy is the most formidable of all, because you don't see him or her coming. This enemy manipulates you from within and inevitably leads you to failure.

Once you've gained control of this enemy within, you can regain control of your life and your weight. But the only way to gain this control is to take the time to analyze your thoughts and behaviours. You have to work on your own self.

But, this takes time and courage. This is a job for heroes. Will you do the work that is needed to become one?

06
OUT WITH THE OLD
AND IN WITH THE NEW

In the example presented in the last chapter, I asked my client to choose between staying obese or doing what was needed to lose weight. If he wants to achieve his goal, he has to change his lifestyle. Thus, for the rest of his life, he will have to learn, apply and repeat the behaviours that will enable him to achieve and maintain a healthy weight. Acting otherwise is tantamount to lying to himself and experiencing failure upon failure.

Although miracle diets and high-intensity exercise have been popular for way too long, weight loss must be achieved by finding a balanced life. There is absolutely no point in starving yourself and training yourself to exhaustion to lose weight. You just need a balanced life.

You must accept the fact that, to achieve your goal, you will have to acquire a new lifestyle and let go of the old one you've been stubbornly holding onto for all these months or years.

To achieve this, you first have to debunk a few myths. So, miracle diets, food deprivation and high-intensity exercise—none of these work. Yes, some of these things sometimes work in the short term, but never in the long term. What is the real goal in losing weight? You should re-member by now... The real goal is: to achieve a healthy weight and to maintain it for the rest of your life.

Along with miracle diets and high-intensity training comes exhaustion. You think all these sacrifices are worth it? But you've already tested all this. And, where does that leave you today? Back at square one, right?

Here is a short discussion with one of my female clients to illustrate what I mean.

— Denis, I've been running for three months and I can't seem to lose any weight. I don't get it... I love to run and I want to run.

— I don't think you'll like my answer. Do you want to hear it anyway?

— That's what I'm here for.

— I've just tested your fitness level. Even though you've been running for three months, your fitness level is very low and, in addition, you're significantly overweight So, unfortunately, you'll have to forget about running for the time being.

— But Denis, I get in shape by running, I don't understand.

— When you run, what is your heart rate zone?

— 165 to 170 beats per minute.

— You see, your ideal heart rate zone is between 115 to 120 beats per minute, which means that you can walk, but you can't run.

— But Denis, I want to run because I love running!

— What is your main goal: running or losing weight?

— Losing weight!

— Then you have to walk and stay in a heart rate zone of 115 to 120 beats per minute.

— But why can't I lose weight by running?

— Because you're not fit enough and you're carrying around too much weight. You reach a heart rate zone in which you deplete your energy reserves, which generates physiological stress and forces your body to store fat.

— Can I at least run once or twice a week?

— No.

— But I need to run.

— What is your main goal: running or losing weight?

— Losing weight.

— Well then, for the time being, stop thinking that running will make you lose weight and just go for walks instead.

— I have a hard time believing what you're telling me, Denis.

— It's simple. You can choose to continue running without losing weight, or you can try my approach. What'll it be?

— But why are you telling me that I won't lose weight by running?

— Because you've been running for three months and you haven't lost any weight. So, what's your choice?

You realize just how powerful a grip your beliefs have on you, don't you? At this point, you might find it difficult to imagine that consuming enough calories and training at low intensity can make you lose weight. But aren't you here to give your body the balance it needs to finally transform itself?

To win, you must "shed" your false beliefs. And that is a job for heroes.

07
TIME GOES BY

The reality is that time goes by. You look back and see that you've been living with your weight or obesity problem for years. As you look ahead, you can't see how your situation will change.

Losing weight requires that you work on your own self, which is a much more intense task that you can imagine. As difficult as it may be, it is the only pathway to achieving your goal.

You will therefore have to acquire new knowledge, adopt new behaviours and repeat those same behaviours, day after day, for the rest of your life.

This truth is not easy to hear, let alone put into practice. My goal is to offer you the tools to get there. All this requires some time and effort on your part.

In five years, will you have the same weight or obesity problems? What about the last five or ten years? Take a look back... and now look ahead. Time goes by. Isn't it time to find a balance in your life that will enable you to achieve a healthy weight and maintain it for the rest of your life?

Time goes by so quickly. Losing weight is a reflection of your life. Make it be fantastic. Losing weight is truly a journey for heroes.

08

READY TO DO WHAT IT TAKES AND ACCEPT REALITY TO LOSE WEIGHT ONCE AND FOR ALL?

Are you still ready to do what it takes to lose weight? Did I hear that right? You said "YES!" Well, let me first let you in on a few unfortunate truths that you will have to face or accept:

- You won't lose weight quickly (between 0.5 lb [200 grams] and 1.25 lb [570 grams] per week for women and between 1 lb [450 grams] and 1.5 lb [680 grams] per week for men).

- You will have to acquire and maintain new lifestyle habits for the rest of your life. Therefore, things won't happen by themselves.

- You will have to challenge your own thoughts and behaviours in order to stop finding excuses to "give yourself permission" to fall back into your old lifestyle habits. You know, the ones that led you down the path to where you are now.

If you accept these truths, you will face them effectively. Your transformation will not happen overnight. It will materialize gradually. You will first set a solid foundation upon which you can build your success. You will encounter difficulties, but you will have the knowledge you need to find the right solution.

Once you've achieved your goal, you won't be the same person. Losing weight is a colossal undertaking. In the end, you will realize that achieving your healthy weight and maintaining it for the rest of your life will be an outstanding life achievement.

Losing weight the smart way, now that's for heroes.

09
THE END IS NEVER THE END

What is your weight loss goal? 15 lb [7 kg], 25 lb [11 kg], 40 lb [18 kg] or 60 lb [27 kg]?[1] How many? Wrong answer... Your goal is to achieve a healthy weight and maintain it for the rest of your life.

Yes, that will translate to a number on your scale, but therein lies a problem. If your goal in your mind is to hit a certain reading on the scale, once you reach that number, like many people, you'll go "YAY! I've finally achieved my goal, my burden is finally over." Do you want to know the harsh reality? Achieving your healthy weight is only the beginning. For the rest of your life, you will have to maintain the behaviours that led you to this success.

The chapters that follow will explain how to set up your plan. The plan itself is meaningless if you don't put it into practice. The plan is basically a set of strategies that must be applied in the form of behaviours to carry out. Behaviours that will yield results over the long term.

Repeating these behaviours every day for the rest of your life means that you will exploit the strengths of your new lifestyle. Put an end to these behaviours and your results will vanish quickly.

The end is never the end. This is the implacable truth, the real cost of achieving your healthy weight and maintaining it for the rest of your life.

Losing weight is truly for heroes.

---

1.   1 kg = 2.2 lb

10
SO, DO YOU STILL WANT TO BECOME A HERO?

One of my clients, who was morbidly obese (51% of his body weight was fat), worked for a major company.

Here is a summary of our conversations.

— Denis, it's time for me do something. My health is deteriorating and I'm only 38 years old.

— Very well then, let's take the necessary steps for you to improve your health.

— Yes, I agree. So what do I have to do?

— OK, I just assessed your metabolism and I will ask you to fill out a daily food diary so that I can follow your progress. You will also have to do three 25-minute light-intensity cardio exercise sessions per week.

— Wow, Denis, that's sounds like a big time commitment!

— What do you think is so time consuming?

— Well, filling out the food diary, 25 minutes of cardio three times a week, coming over here to meet with you, etc.

— So, what is the purpose of coming to see me?

— Like I said, Denis, I want to lose weight.

— All right, but who do you think has to do the work?

— I know I do, Denis, but I work for a very important company and I also have a very important job.

— Well then that's great! We have our answer.

— The answer to what? I don't get it...

— It's very simple, you're going to fail.

— What? How can you say I'm going to fail?

— My years of experience. In fact, you just alluded to the fact that your work is your most important value. Before even taking the first step to improve your health, you just told me that your work will always come before your health.

— No Denis, that's not what I meant to say.

— Regardless of what you may say, your actions will speak louder than words. You will continue to hold onto your current lifestyle habits and you are nowhere near changing any of them because you haven't done the necessary work to be able to change that lifestyle.

Once again, I know what you're thinking: "What a deplorable attitude. Doesn't he want to take control of his own health?" Really? Think about it for a second: are you all that different? How many times in your life have you chosen to invest time in all kinds of activities other than those that could have had benefits for your health? If your reply is something along the lines of "Yes, that's happened to me, Denis. But I was short of time. A lot of things happened to me and I just didn't have enough time to take care of myself," then tell me how are you any different from my client?

Just think about when someone arrives late for a meeting and you say "that guy can never be on time," yet, when YOU are late for a meeting you say: "Sorry I'm late, it's not my fault, I got stuck in traffic."

Losing weight is for people who hold their health as a top priority. No excuses. Only action. I repeat: No excuses...

Losing weight is truly for heroes.

11
I'VE TRULY ACCEPTED

I can feel it. You're ready for another little summary/discussion.

First month

— Denis, I truly realize now that losing weight takes the time it takes. I'm shooting for slow but steady weight loss. In the last three years, I haven't lost a pound. It's time for me to do something different.

— Very well then. Take the next month to implement your program. Don't pressure yourself. You won't achieve perfection. Take the time to understand the process. Based on your results, I think you will lose weight at a rate of three-quarters of a pound (340 grams) per week.

— I'm going for it. I'm changing my lifestyle.

Second month

— This is better than I expected. You've lost 5 lb in one month. Congratulations!

— Ummm....

— What's this "Ummm...?"

— Well, to be perfectly honest, I'm a little disappointed because I expected better results.

— OK… So what happened to this epiphany you reported to me that made you realize that losing weight would take the time it takes? Do you remember our discussion at our first meeting?

— Yeah, I know, but it's still a bit disappointing.

— What's disappointing?

— I was hoping to lose 7 lb in the first month.

— And so these 5 lb you lost are a failure to you. At our first meeting, to whom were you lying, me or yourself?

There can sometimes be a considerable gap between stating your acceptance of a situation and really accepting it when you are actually faced with it.

If you are undertaking this process but that, "deep down," you want to lose weight quickly, you will fail. Don't kid yourself. Today, you are undertaking a long-term process that involves a lifestyle change, along with a slow, healthy weight loss.

True weight loss means losing weight for good. And that, my friends, is for heroes.

12

LOSING WEIGHT THE SMART WAY ONCE AND FOR ALL

Do you see? Losing weight is a personal journey. A journey for heroes.

What is your choice, for you, right now? Whatever you choose, make that choice, and accept the consequences.

Losing weight is for heroes, those who progress, evolve, transform themselves from within and adopt effective behaviours, without any resentment, for the rest of their lives.

You can also choose to continue to eat and drink as much as you want. If you choose to continue down this road, however, be prepared to live with the consequences: extra weight or obesity.

There are no "middle-ground" solutions.

Losing weight is for heroes who make the necessary choices to achieve their goals. Their reward: losing weight the smart way once and for all.

PART 2
INITIATING THE WEIGHT LOSS PROCESS

13
SETTING THE FOUNDATIONS

Well, here you are! You are about to embark on this heroic journey. The time has come to implement your program. The following chapters will guide you step by step.

Take the time to read, to think, and reread each chapter as often as you need. Remind yourself that I'm inviting you to acquire new knowledge, which will lead you to adopt new behaviours that you will have to incorporate into your life in the months ahead. All of this takes time, patience and reflection.

This will not be an easy task. Many difficulties lie ahead But you will be well equipped to face these challenges. This will only make your victory that much more gratifying.

Losing weight is for heroes.

14
CHANGING YOUR BELIEFS

A belief is an idea we have about how the world, a situation, a thing or an event works.

A belief is therefore a "truth" that we hold as immutable because we maintain it in our thoughts. And since our thoughts are our own, we rarely call them into question.

As I will explain later on, weight loss is based on the functioning of your metabolism and how it distributes and uses your body's energy reserves. Unfortunately, weight loss has for decades been viewed from a strictly mathematical perspective.

Thus, as one pound of fat (450 grams) contains 3,500 calories of energy, it is therefore considered that spending (through exercise) or reducing one's caloric intake by 3,500 calories will result in the loss of one pound (450 grams) of fat.

You have therefore been "sold" this concept of weight loss in every which way possible by your mother, your father, a cousin, friends, ads, miracle diet and program promotions, etc. And this belief is very deeply entrenched in your mind. You believe it so much that you cannot even imagine that weight loss may work differently.

This mathematical model of weight loss that is so deeply rooted in people's minds to the point of becoming a popular belief has led to aberrant behaviour. This belief leads you to spend (through exercise) the highest possible number of calories and to reduce your caloric intake as much as possible.

In short, to meet the requirements of this belief, you train to exhaustion and constantly suffer from starvation.

If this mathematical model of weight loss (belief) really worked, you wouldn't be reading this book. Yes, in the short term, you will see some weight loss using this model. However, since your body is pushed into a situation of physiological stress, after a few weeks, your metabolism will slow down in order to spend as few calories as possible. It will also store more fat in order to generate energy reserves, in the event that you would imperil your body for a long period of time.

In order to reject this belief and initiate a balanced weight loss process, one that will not subject your body to physiological stress, you have to understand that gaining and losing weight depends on the regulation of your nervous system and your hormonal system. And there is nothing mathematical when it comes to these systems. This is a completely different world where calories (energy available to your metabolism) are chemical energy units that will be directed to the fat storage zone (your fat cells) or your liver (important energy reserve management organ) or the production of energy (muscular work and heat production). When your body is in a state of balance, it directs its energy reserves mainly to the liver and muscles and you lose weight. Subject your body to physiological stress and it will direct the energy to the storage zone, and you gain weight.

Consider this example. Your basal metabolic rate is 1,400 calories. You follow a diet of 1,200 calories (200 calories fewer than your basal metabolism requires) for one month and you train 5 times a week, where you spend 800 calories at each training session. On average, you have a daily deficit of 1,000 (200 + 800) calories per day. According to the mathematical model of weight loss (belief), you should lose 2 lb per week, every week, non-stop.

But is that what really happens? Of course not! Inevitably, as your caloric intake is clearly lower than what your basal metabolism requires and that you are training to exhaustion, your nervous system and your hormonal system team up to protect you against your own self. Your basal metabolic rate will slow down to reduce your energy expenditure and more of the calories you consume will be directed to the storage zone (fat cells).

All that effort for so little gain.

As you read the next few chapters, you will gain a better understanding of how your metabolism works. You will think: "Yes, it all makes perfect sense," but in reality, as you will be eating your fill and doing moderate exercise, you will initially have a hard time believing that you can lose weight with such little effort. Your old die-hard belief will make you want to starve yourself and train to exhaustion once again. This will trouble your mind for a while. Just one piece of advice: Resist! Never go back to repeating those old mistakes that never worked.

Give yourself some time to let this new knowledge sink in. Once you start seeing results, you will finally see weight loss from a completely different angle.

Losing weight also requires that you change the way you think. And, once again, that's a job for heroes.

15
YOUR KNOWLEDGE ABOUT METABOLIC FUNCTIONING

How about another summary of a discussion with a client?

— Denis, I've been following the program for a month, and it's really weird. I eat my fill and I don't sweat a drop when I train and I've lost 6 lb. I'm ready to step things up a notch.

— What do you mean by "step things up a notch?"

— I figure it's time to push myself a bit more and train at a higher intensity...

— Really? Why?

— Because I want to spend more calories and lose weight faster.

— Are you sure about that?

— And while we're at it, since I have a hard time eating all of the recommended 1,600 calories every day, could I reduce my caloric intake?

— OK, let's go over all this together. In the last month, you ate your fill, namely 1,600 calories per day. Doing low-intensity exercise has now become easy for you to do and is now a fun part of your life's routine. Thanks to that, you just melted away 6 lb of fat, and now you want to go back to your old ways of doing things... And If I remember well, you told me at our first meeting that you had deprived yourself and trained at high intensity for three years without shedding a single pound.

How many times do you think I've heard these types of comments? Dozens of times. The mathematical model of weight loss (belief) is so deeply entrenched in human brains that it makes it difficult to accept the fact that giving your body a balanced life (consuming enough calories and training at low intensity) will result in weight loss.

Your body transforms itself when it is in a state of equilibrium and not when it is subjected to physiological stress (deprivation and high-intensity exercise).

Here are two fundamental questions:

- Why do we have to eat to lose weight?
- How does low-intensity training burn fat?

Why do we have to eat to lose weight? The answer is simple: because if you consume fewer calories than your basal metabolic rate requires, your metabolism will slow down and your body will begin to store more fat.

Small definition: The basal metabolic rate is the amount of energy required for every cell in your body (your skin, your brain, your heart, your kidneys, your liver, your bones, your muscles, etc.) can do its work while you are at rest.

If you have a basal metabolic rate of 1,500 calories per day, this means that your body requires 1,500 calories for all of your cells to do their job. And this does not take into account the calories you spend at work and during exercise.

Therefore, if your basal metabolic rate is 1,500 calories and you only consume 1,200 calories in the hope of losing weight, your metabolism will work to slow down to nearly 1,200 calories. Why? Because that is the amount of energy made available to your body. Yes, you'll lose weight in the first weeks, but your body will end up resisting the weight loss by slowing its metabolism and storing more fat.

Once your body starts resisting the weight loss, no matter how much you fight it, your body will win because it must survive (by storing fat).

In order for you to win over your body and get it to burn fat once again, you have to provide it with the balance in needs.

This balance is the only tool that leads to weight loss.

Losing weight is for people who can accept that "balance" is clearly more effective in the long term, realizing at the same time that there is nothing spectacular about this fact.

Losing weight is for heroes.

16
YOUR HEALTHY WEIGHT

If you poke around on the Internet, you can find some kind of formula to calculate your healthy weight. Most of the time, however, the "healthy weight" that is suggested to you makes no sense. In fact, it is impossible to achieve in most cases. Why is that? Because the calculation does not take into account your body composition.

What is body composition? It is your total weight defined in terms of the proportion of lean mass (muscles, bones, internal organs) and fat mass.

Let's consider the example of two women. A healthy weight for women varies between 28% and 32% fat. Thus, 28% to 32% of the body's weight is made up of fat. For men, 20% to 24% fat represents a healthy weight.

Both of our women are of equal height and weigh 180.4 lb [82 kg]. However, their body compositions are very different:

Woman 1

Total weight: 180.4 lb [82 kg]
Lean mass: 116.6 lb [53 kg]
Fat mass: 63.8 lb [29 kg]
Percentage of fat: 35.4% (63.8 ÷ 180.4 or 29 ÷ 82)

Therefore, 35.4% of this woman's body is made up of fat.

Woman 2

Total weight: 180.4 lb [82 kg]
Lean mass: 99 lb [45 kg]
Fat mass: 81.4 lb [37 kg]
Percentage of fat: 45% (81.4 ÷ 180.4 or 37 ÷ 82)

Therefore, 45% of this woman's body is made up of fat.

Let's imagine now that each of these two women would like to achieve a healthy weight with 28% body fat.

Woman 1

She would need to lose 18.5 lb [8.4 kg].

Woman 2

She would need to lose 43 lb [19.5 kg].

I've illustrated a pretty significant difference between these women's lean mass to help you understand the fact that lean mass is an important determining factor in the measurement of a healthy weight.

Thus, the Body Mass Index (BMI) is not a very good indicator of your healthy weight, as it does not take into account your lean mass.

A bioimpedance scale is a very good investment if you want to follow the evolution of your weight.

Here is another example: You've lost 5 lb (2.2 kg) of fat and gained 3 lb (1.4 kg) of lean mass (muscle). A regular scale will indicate that you've only lost 2 lb (900 grams), whereas a bioimpedance scale will clearly indicate that you've lost 5 lb (2.2 kg) of fat and gained 3 lb (1.4 kg) of lean mass.

Here is an example to help you do the calculations if your bioimpedance scale doesn't give you all the details.

Scale reading 1

Weight: 90 kg (198 lb)
Percentage of fat: 42%
Fat mass: 37.8 kg [(42 X 90) ÷ 100]
Lean mass: 52.2 kg [90 kg (total weight) − 37.8 (fat mass)]

Scale reading 2

Weight: 88 kg (193.6)
Fat mass: 35.6 kg (loss of 2.2 kg)
Lean mass: 53.6 kg (gain of 1.4 kg)
Percentage of fat: 40.5% (35.6 ÷ 88)

In this example, the person's total weight only decreased by 2 kg (4.4 lb), but the loss of 2.2 kg (4.84) of fat and the gain of 1.4 kg (3.1 lb) of lean mass mean that the percentage of fat dropped from 42% to 40.5%.

If you can afford it, purchase a bioimpedance scale. Keep in mind, however, that they are very sensitive to your hydration level, which can cause significant variations in the lean mass and fat mass values. I recommend that you take scale readings at the same time of the day, on an empty stomach and without having consumed any liquids for approximately 2 hours.

17
STAY CALM, RELAXED, AND READ AGAIN

The following chapters will explain how to implement your weight loss program. This is the most technical part of the program.

Take the time to read and assimilate all of the information. Go at it at your own pace; it's not a race against time.

Faced with so much information, many people get discouraged at the first reading. I'll say it again: Take your time, read, and read again, until everything makes sense in your mind. Stay calm, relaxed, and read. Stay calm, relaxed, and read again. Stay calm, relaxed, and... read as often as necessary.

This way, you will eventually develop the knowledge and strategies that will enable you to progress throughout your hero's journey.

Losing weight is for heroes who invest the time to succeed.

18
DETERMINING YOUR
BASAL METABOLIC RATE

Your basal metabolic rate can be evaluated using any of three methods, but their accuracy varies. Since you're reading this book, only one of these methods is available to you for the time being.

The most accurate method involves the use, as I do in the lab, of a respiratory gas analyzer. This device is used to measure your oxygen consumption and how your body burns lipids and carbohydrates. Given that one litre of oxygen consumed represents an expenditure of 5 calories, your caloric expenditure (basal metabolic rate) can then easily be determined. Although this method is the most accurate, it does carry a certain margin of error, as your metabolism is not necessarily stable at all times. This is especially true for women. This means that I must subject my female clients to repeated tests in order to obtain a satisfactory measurement of their basal metabolic rate. There may be a laboratory in your area that can provide this service.

The second method can be used to estimate your basal metabolic rate by taking into account your body composition. Given that your lean mass (muscles, bones, internal organs) are the main determinants of your basal metabolic rate, once your lean mass is known, calculation formulas can be used to determine your basal metabolic rate. A bioimpedance scale is the best tool to determine your body composition (total weight, lean mass, fat mass).

Lastly, as you are reading this book, only the third method is available to you: the Harris and Benedict Equation, which is one of the better-known formulas to calculate the basal metabolic rate (Harris J, Benedict F. A biometric study of basal metabolism in man. Washington D.C. Carnegie Institute of Washington. 1919.), which, as you can see, goes all the way back to 1919. Not to worry, however, it's validity remains very good for people who have good nutrition, but it has a margin of error of plus or minus 14%.

Equation for women

Basal metabolic rate = 655 + (9.6 x your weight in kg)
+ (1.8 X your height in cm) – (4.7 x your age).

Equation for men

Basal metabolic rate = 66 + (13.7 x your weight in kg)
+ (5 x your height in cm) – (6.8 x your age).

Regardless of the method you use, remember that your metabolism (especially among women) varies constantly and is affected by several factors (your state of health), situations or events (stress). We rarely get a 100% accurate measurement. There will always be a margin of error with any method used.

Now that you know the number of calories you spend at rest every day (your basal metabolic rate), you can determine your daily caloric intake.

19

DETERMINING YOUR DAILY CALORIC INTAKE

At rest, while sitting or lying down, your energy expenditure is called your basal metabolic rate.

However, as soon as you get up, walk, do the dishes, go up the stairs, work on the computer, drive your car, exercise, etc., you spend more calories than you do at rest.

This is therefore an additional caloric expenditure. A simple way to estimate your caloric expenditure is to multiply your basal metabolic rate (which you evaluated in the preceding chapter) by one of the factors presented in the following table.

Once again, this is an estimate, but it will give you a good idea of your energy expenditure during activity.

To measure your caloric expenditure during activity, you simply need to determine whether you are sedentary, mildly active, moderately active, active or very active and select the factor (see the following table) that corresponds to your level of activity and then multiply your basal metabolic rate by this factor.

**MULTIPLICATON FACTOR ASSOCIATED
WITH LEVEL OF PHYSICAL ACTIVITY**

Level of Activity	Factor
Sedentary	1.1
Mildly active (30 to 45 minutes of light exercise per day)	1.15
Moderately active (45 minutes to 1 hour of moderate-intensity exercise 4 to 5 hours per week)	1.2
Active (5 to 8 hours of training per week)	1.3
Very active (more than 8 hours of training per week, including work of a physical nature in which you are in constant movement)	1.8

If you want to perform more precise calculations concerning your energy expenditure, you can use a number of online tools that are available free of charge for this purpose.

Calculating your total energy expenditure

Now, to find out how many calories you spend in total every day (basal metabolic rate and caloric expenditure during activity), you simply have to multiply your basal metabolic rate by the factor that corresponds to your level of activity.

Thus, if you evaluated your basal metabolic rate at 1,450 calories and your level of activity at "moderately active," just multiply 1,450 by 1.2 for a total of 1,740 calories spent per day. From these 1,740 calories, 1,450 are attributable to your basal metabolic rate, and 290 (1,740 - 1,450) to the additional energy expenditure from your daily activities.

I insist once again on the importance of consuming the number of calories that are necessary for your basal metabolism to function effectively. In this case, with a basal metabolic rate of 1,450 calories, I suggest consuming between 1,450 and 1,500 calories.

Ah yes, I can hear the panic set in. "But Denis, that makes no sense! You suggest consuming more calories than the basal metabolic rate. I'll gain weight!" No you won't. Forget the mathematical weight loss model (belief). In this example, I'm adding 50 calories to the basal metabolic rate (1,450 + 50) to meet the energy requirements (calories) of the basal metabolic rate and a portion of the requirements associated with daily activities (housekeeping, doing the dishes, getting up, walking a little bit, etc.). This strategy aims to ensure that your body is never in an energy deficit (or surplus, of course). This will help distribute your energy reserves effectively. Your body is now in the ideal situation to burn fat.

Once again, I know what you're thinking: "But Denis, where is the caloric deficit that will enable me to lose weight?" Remember, you're no longer seeking to achieve a caloric deficit, but rather a proper metabolic balance. You no longer operate on the basis of the mathematical model of weight loss, but rather on the model of energy reserve distribution.

The energy reserve distribution model implies that when your nutrition meets the needs of your basal metabolism, more energy is directed toward the liver (a very important organ in the management of energy reserves) and the muscles, and less toward the storage zone (fat cells). Furthermore, in a state of metabolic equilibrium, your fat cells release the stored fat more easily to be burned by your cells (muscles and other organs that need energy). And there you have it: your metabolism is working at maximum efficiency. A bit later, I will explain how exercise can improve the functioning of your metabolism.

What happens now if you spend many calories during training? Let's imagine that you're a very active person. I multiply your basal metabolic rate (1,450 calories in our example) by the factor of 1.8, which gives an expenditure of 2,610 calories in your day.

I can hear you panic once again: "Denis, are you telling me I have to consume 2,610 calories? Are you crazy?" No, I'm not crazy. This is simply the logic that results from energy reserve distribution.

Here is the golden rule to remember: Never consume fewer calories than your basal metabolic rate, and if you spend many calories during work or exercise, maintain a maximum deficit of 400 calories.

In the last example, the expenditure is 2,610 calories, from which I subtract 400 calories (maximum deficit), which means that the person should consume approximately 2,210 calories.

The multiplication factor associated with the level of activity also carries a margin of error. Several activity monitors (Fitbit, Polar, Garmin, Timex, etc.) also give you an indication of your energy expenditure. However, it is impossible to get a perfectly accurate reading from any of these methods. There will always be a margin of error and, in many cases, activity monitors fairly significantly overestimate energy expenditure.

To obtain a more precise measurement of your energy expenditure, you can use a number of online tools that are available free of charge for this purpose.

Distribution of proteins, lipids and carbohydrates

In order to function properly, your body needs proteins, lipids and carbohydrates. For a weight loss program, I recommend that you distribute your intake of proteins, lipids and carbohydrates as follows:

- 25% of your total caloric intake in proteins.
- 40% of your total caloric intake in lipids.
- 35% of your total caloric intake in carbohydrates.

This distribution corresponds to the needs of 70% of the population.

Before we perform a more concrete calculation, it is important that you remember the following:

- One gram of proteins contains four calories.
- One gram of carbohydrates contains four calories.
- One gram of lipids (fat) contains nine calories.

This distribution varies from one person to another based on the evaluation of their basal metabolic rate and type of training. For me, however, this distribution constitutes a central value around which I apply variations.

In this example, I'm using 1,500 calories as the daily caloric intake. This is just an example, not the norm. I have clients who measure 1.90 m with an impressive muscle mass and a metabolism of 3,100 calories. They lose weight with a caloric intake of 3,500 calories per day...

I supervise athletes that must consume 6,000 calories per day to meet their energy requirements.

To each his own metabolism; to each his own caloric intake.

Here is an example of the distribution of proteins, lipids and carbohydrates for a caloric intake of 1,500 calories:

- Proteins: 25% of the total caloric intake (1,500 calories), namely 375 calories or 94 grams.
- Lipids: 40% of the total caloric intake, namely 600 calories or 67 grams.
- Carbohydrates: 35% of the total caloric intake, namely 525 calories or 131 grams.

This distribution will have to be rectified, however, once you have reached the maintenance stage. Once my clients have reached this stage, I usually recommend that they go back to a carbohydrate intake of 40% to 45% of the total caloric intake and to slightly reduce the proteins and lipids. Once again, these values vary from one person to another. In this book, I can only provide a central tendency of functioning.

20
FILLING OUT YOUR FOOD DIARY

Now that you've just completed all of these wonderful calculations, what do you have to do? Get an accurate idea of the value of the foods you consume to make sure you get as close as possible to the maximum recommended values (calories, proteins, lipids, carbohydrates). Remember, however, that you will never reach 100% of these values at any time. A variation of 5% is both acceptable and normal.

Once again, to make your life easier, I invite you to use online tools that are available free of charge for this purpose.

I know what you're thinking: "Denis, are you telling me that I have to weigh all of my food and enter everything I eat and drink in a food diary?" That's exactly what I'm saying! How else can you know whether what you consume matches the calculations you just completed? You can't go into this blindly. Furthermore, what is the point of undertaking this program if you don't want to invest the time required to understand your nutrition?

I strongly recommend that you fill out your food diary every day for the first month. This is the only way you'll acquire the knowledge you need about your nutrition. After that, I recommend that you fill it out at least 4 days a week (including a Saturday or Sunday) for the next 12 months. No excuses... You really want to succeed, so do it!

21
UNDERTAKING YOUR CARDIO PROGRAM

In your opinion, which training program will be the most effective?

1. Training at high intensity 5 days a week, 90 minutes per session and then quitting after 2 months.

2. Training at low intensity for an hour and a half to two hours per week divided into short 15- to 20-minute sessions for the rest of your life.

Although option 2 is the least impressive, it is the most effective.

— Denis, I didn't train last month because I couldn't meet my training goals.

— What exactly are these "training goals" you speak of?

— Well, to achieve results, I have to train 5 to 6 hours a week.

— Hold on a second. Do you remember the initial program in which I asked you to train 90 to 120 minutes per week? Do you also remember that you lost a lot of weight by following this program?

— Well, Denis, I want even better results and I'm shooting for 5 to 6 hours of training per week. Since I wasn't able to do that because of my work, I just didn't bother training.

— All right, but tell me. During this intense work period, could you have done 6 training sessions of 15 minutes each per week?

— Of course!

— Let me sum it up. Since you couldn't train 5 to 6 hours a week, you didn't train at all... So, "zero" training. But, you would have had time to do 6 training sessions of 15 minutes each for a total of 90 minutes a week. What do you think is the most effective in the long run: 90 minutes of training per week for the rest of your life, or "zero" training for the rest of your life?

Yes indeed, I assure you, I've had this type of discussion with some of my clients. Don't think they are the only ones to hold onto such ineffective beliefs. The oddness of their behaviour becomes really obvious when you read the transcript of our discussion but, in reality, it is quite likely that you may also behave that way yourselves.

Disproportionate training goals (in terms of both intensity and duration) are, in most cases, irreconcilable with everyday life. Family, work, leisure, etc. all demand time. And time, unfortunately, is a limited resource.

Before undertaking your training program, I invite you to think about the actual time you can free up every week. For now, don't think about any minimum number of hours you need to achieve results. Think and check off your answer:

- ❏ 2 sessions of 20 minutes per week.
- ❏ 2 sessions of 30 minutes per week.
- ❏ 4 sessions of 15 minutes per week.
- ❏ 3 sessions of 30 minutes per week.
- ❏ 6 sessions of 15 minutes per week.
- ❏ 4 sessions of 30 minutes per week.
- ❏ 2 sessions of 1 hour per week.
- ❏ 6 sessions of 30 minutes per week.
- ❏ 3 sessions of 1 hour per week.

Now, let's take a look at the cardio program. The goal of the cardio program is to enable you to use the heart rate zone in which you will burn the most fat to produce the energy your body requires. This represents light- to moderate-intensity effort.

Once again, I can hear you thinking: "But Denis, if I train within a light- to moderate-intensity zone, I won't spend many calories." Remember, you're no longer using the mathematical model of weight loss (belief); you are exploiting the strengths of the energy reserve distribution model.

Contrary to what you may think, by targeting the heart rate zone in which you burn the most fat, you are stimulating your body in the most efficient manner possible to lose weight. I often say that high-intensity exercise is a scam. Why is that? Carefully read what follows.

The data listed in the table below are from energy expenditure under effort tests that I conducted in my exercise physiology lab.

In the left-hand column, I list the zone and the fuel you are burning (lipids or carbohydrates). The aerobic zone enables you to burn lipids (fat) and the anaerobic zone burns carbohydrates.

CALORIC EXPENDITURE UNDER EFFORT

Zones/ Fuel/ Intensity	Caloric Expenditure/Minute		
	Sedentary	Active	Fit
Aerobic/Lipids/Light to moderate	7	9	14
Aerobic/Carbohydrates/ Extreme or maximum	11	14	19
Difference	4	5	5

For a sedentary individual, the heart rate zone in which the maximum amount of lipids are burned involves an expenditure of 7 calories per minute. At maximum effort, in which the maximum amount of carbohydrates are burned (thereby totally exhausting your energy reserves), the expenditure is 11 calories per minute. The difference is only 4 calories.

In short, if a sedentary individual does a 30-minute cardio session by respecting the heart rate zone in which he or she burns the most fat, this person will spend 210 calories (30 minutes X 7 calories/minute). If, by some miracle, this person were to manage to train to his or her maximum capacity (which is impossible to maintain over this long a period and hazardous to the person's health) for 30 minutes, he or she would spend 330 calories (30 minutes X 11 calories). Therefore, exhausting yourself through maximum intensity exercise only burns 120 more calories than a low intensity session (heart rate zone in which you burn the most lipids). And remember, this calculation only applies to a case where the person maintains maximum effort for a solid 30 minutes. Does it finally shed this pointless "need" to push yourself to the limit every time you train?

To help you identify the heart rate zone in which you burn the most fat, you can use the effort intensity perception scale presented in the figure below as a guide.

Here, "0" indicates no effort and "10" indicates maximum effort.

Your maximal fat oxidation zone is between "2" and "4." You should also know that during effort you perceive as very easy, namely "1" (e.g. walking slowly), you are still burning fat.

INTENSITY EFFORT PERCEPTION SCALE

0	1	2	3	4	5	6	7	8	9	10
Nothing at all	Very easy	Easy	Average	Somewhat difficult	Difficult	More difficult	Very difficult	Very, very difficult	Extremely difficult	Maximum

Yes, even when you walk slowly, you are burning fat. Furthermore, regardless of whether you walk or run 10 km, you spend the same number of calories. So then, what's the point of exhausting yourself when you can walk slowly over a given distance and spend as many calories as if you were running, burning fat the whole time? Yes indeed, you can lose weight without exhausting yourself.

Now that you've identified the heart rate zone in which you burn the most fat, it's up to you to lace up those sneakers and strap on your heart rate monitor to follow the evolution of your heart rate to make sure you are respecting YOUR heart rate zone. Then, you only have to dedicate the time (for the rest of your life) you have available every week to train, as you determined above. So is it...

- ❏ 2 sessions of 20 minutes per week.
- ❏ 2 sessions of 30 minutes per week.
- ❏ 4 sessions of 15 minutes per week.
- ❏ 3 sessions of 30 minutes per week.
- ❏ 6 sessions of 15 minutes per week.
- ❏ 4 sessions of 30 minutes per week.
- ❏ 2 sessions of 1 hour per week.
- ❏ 6 sessions of 30 minutes per week.
- ❏ 3 sessions of 1 hour per week.

Muscle training

Science now considers the muscles as the largest internal organ of the human body with the capacity to communicate with other organs such as the brain, the liver, and fat cells, through the secretion of hormones.

Muscle stimulation through training therefore fosters the secretion of hormones that allow lipids to be released from fat cells to then be used by the body.

Once again, to use the muscles' "communication" properties, it is not necessary to train to your muscles' maximum capacity. A regular and well-paced training program will enable you to achieve your goals better than a high-intensity muscle training program that will generate stress on your body and a risk of injury.

There is such a wide variety of muscle training programs out there that I recommend you consult a private trainer (preferably with a university degree in the field) to develop a customized program that is adapted to your capacities.

When you ask a trainer to teach you a program, explain that you don't want to exhaust yourself, nor do you want to have to exert excessive effort. Mention to this person that you want a program that will stimulate your muscles without driving you to exhaustion. I emphasize this point because too many trainers still believe that a training program is only effective when the person is pushed to the limit of his or her capacities.

22

MANAGING YOUR BEHAVIOUR AND YOUR WEIGHT LOSS

You now have the tools you need to undertake your weight loss program. You've just put down the solid foundations you will need to succeed.

Once again, I know what you're thinking: "This is a total nightmare, Denis. I understand absolutely nothing about all this talk of calories, proteins, lipids, carbohydrates, food diaries, exercise and everything else!" My reply: Stay calm, relaxed and read again. Stay calm, relaxed and... read as often as necessary.

You have to look at your first month as a learning period. Use trial and error. You can't possibly know everything, master everything and do everything perfectly from the word go. You have to give yourself the time to absorb all of the knowledge that is essential to your weight loss plan. Without it, you'll just be headed for failure.

This next comment will be very tough, but several clients tell me that they are perfectionists who want to control the slightest detail to perfection. These clients give up very quickly, as many of them are afraid of failure and point to all of these useless details they couldn't "do perfectly" to justify their inability to move forward. The devil is in the details. Don't make your plan a living hell right from the start.

Usually, the second month is when you'll have much greater control over the knowledge and behaviours you'll have to master... for the rest of your life. For most people, this is when confidence starts to set in.

And then there are those whose vigilance has already started to wane. Just not enough time. Remember? Those who still had not placed their health as a top priority. Go back to your plan constantly and fill out your food diary. Keep going back to the basic behaviours that produce results.

Throughout the weeks ahead, you will progress. However, you will also encounter daily temptations: weekends spent wining and dining with friends, office parties, the holiday season, gluttony, the desire to reward yourself with a little treat, etc. You'll also go through the normal stages in a weight loss process that some see as failure, such as reaching plateaus. Never let this book leave your side. Read it as often as necessary, as it will help remind you of the reason why you are straying, if such is the case.

Achieving your healthy weight must be done as you live your normal life. This is not something you can accomplish outside of your regular life. And, to maintain your healthy weight for the rest of your life, your new behaviours must have generated a new lifestyle for you.

Thus, you will encounter many difficulties. But, knowing that this is normal, and by being well prepared, you will have everything you need to face these situations successfully.

Losing weight is for heroes who transform their lives to give their bodies the necessary balance to achieve its own transformation.

PART 3
FOR THE REST OF YOUR LIFE

23
BUILDING YOUR SUCCESS
ONE BEHAVIOUR AT A TIME

Progress, not perfection... Take your time. Losing weight means achieving a healthy weight and maintaining it for the rest of your life. This is not a sprint race. It's an ultra-marathon. Stay calm, and gradually incorporate the information taught in this book, one behaviour at a time.

— All right Denis, I'll put that into practice as soon as possible. But when can I start the muscle-building program?

— Actually, for the first month, I want you to focus primarily on your nutrition. Take the time to fill out your food diary every day and be sure to gradually incorporate quality foods. Then, start your cardio program as I prescribed.

— So no muscle-building...

— Not for now. For the time being, we need to build a solid foundation and then gradually adjust your cardio and muscle-building program.

— But I feel like I'll be wasting time.

— What time will you be wasting?

— Well, I'd lose weight faster if I started everything at once.

— And why should you do all this as quickly as possible? The important thing is to build your success by incorporating one behaviour at a time. There's nothing easier than tying to apply everything at once and giving up after 2 or 3 weeks.

— Not sure I'm following you, Denis.

— For you to reach your weight loss goals, I'm forcing you, to a certain extent, to adopt a number of new behaviours. It seems easy, but it's actually very difficult and exhausting. However, if you incorporate one behaviour, and you repeat that behaviour over a long enough period of time, it becomes an automatic response. You no longer even have to think about it. Then, you do the same thing with another behaviour until it too becomes automatic. In the end, instead of wearing out your neurons by always thinking about the new behaviours you have to adopt and maintain, you just have to work on one at a time until it becomes an automatic response and, after a few months, all of these behaviours will have become second nature.

Losing weight is for people who do things differently and who give themselves the time they need to learn.

Losing weight is for heroes.

24
YOU'RE GOING TO FORGET, BUT THE SECRET LIES IN THE INITIAL PLAN

Here's another discussion I had with one of my clients to illustrate the subject. As a bonus, my thoughts appear in italics...

We've reached the fourth month. Average weight loss of 4 lb per month. Therefore, a total of 12 lb lost. The goal was to lose 17 lb to reach a healthy weight and to maintain it for the rest of her life.

— Denis, I don't feel like I've lost any weight in the last month.

— Indeed, your weight has remained stable since I weighed you last month. Has anything different happened? Stress, fatigue, insomnia, new medication?

— No, absolutely nothing.

— But I see you're no longer filling out your food diary.

— Did you continue to follow our plan?

— Actually, I stopped filling out my food diary because I'm sure I'm following our plan.

— *Here's yet another client who no longer quantifies anything and thinks she's still on target.* Then how do you know if you're still respecting the proper distribution of calories, proteins, lipids and carbohydrates?

— I think I'm pretty accurate...

— *I think...* OK, let's say you are. So if your nutrition is fine, how then do you explain the fact that you didn't lose any weight?

— I have no idea. Maybe I should train harder?

— *And here it is... The truth is just around the corner.* So, you still think that you have to train a lot and at high intensity to lose weight?

— Well, I figure my body must eventually get used to low-intensity exercise, and maybe that's why I stopped losing weight

— *She's decided to do it her way.* And in the last month, did you follow the training plan to the letter, or did you do more than prescribed?

— Well, I went from 3 cardio sessions of 30 minutes each at 130 beats per minute to 5 sessions of 45 minutes each at 150 beats per minute.

— *There is no worse blind person than the one who doesn't want to see.* That's really impressive. You followed the plan to the letter for the first 3 months and you lost 12 of the 17 pounds we had set as a goal. You had proof that the plan was working perfectly and, now that you've gone back to your old beliefs and habits, you've stopped losing weight. When you first came to see me three months ago, didn't we determine that you weren't losing weight because you were training too much?

— Um... yeah...

— Then why in the world would you want to go back to the strategy that prevented you from losing weight?

There you go folks. Despite the evidence, you will eventually stray from the right path. This is why your plan needs to be written down in black and white. This way, when you get off track, you can get back to the original plan. The one that really works. Not the one you believe, not the one that should work, not the one you would like to see produce results. No, the one written down in black and white that really works.

Losing weight is for those who tirelessly follow, without changing, a plan that has proven its effectiveness. Others get lost in the details and lose sight of the main point.

Losing weight is for those who don't get lost in conjecture. Losing weight is for heroes.

25
ONE DAY, YOU WILL HAVE TO STOP LOSING WEIGHT

When I explain to my clients that once they've reached their healthy weight, they will then have to enter the maintenance stage, I see this weird reaction in their eyes that says something like: "Really? I'll have to stop losing weight one day? I'd never thought of that."

In my opinion, this reaction merely reflects repeated failures. Over the years, you've lost weight many times only to eventually gain it all back again that, for a big part of your life, all you've thought about was losing weight. You never realized that, one day, you could be completely free from this burden.

Therefore, you will lose weight, you will reach a healthy weight, and you will enter a maintenance stage. Which means that you will never again have to think about losing weight. However, for the rest of your life, you will have to act in ways that will allow you to maintain your healthy weight. Fortunately, you've just incorporated new habits into your life. You have an effective plan that has given you confidence in yourself.

You are finally in control of your life.

Losing weight is for the hero you are in the process of becoming.

26
BUT, THERE WILL BE A CRITICAL MOMENT WHEN EVERYTHING COULD FALL APART

Your process will follow a cycle: the initial motivation that led you to read this book and apply the strategies presented within; the time and effort you've invested; the confrontations with yourself; assimilating new knowledge and behaviours; your body's transformations; your vigilance as you face hazards and temptations; the benefits of losing weight; satisfaction with your results; confidence that everything will be fine; satisfaction with success; and... easing off.

Remember, the end is not the end. As a result of this cycle you will go through, easing off is that extremely dangerous time when you think that you've achieved all your goals and that you can now do whatever you want.

What a joy it is to be able to take advantage of your success, this feeling of achievement and freedom, and the wonderful feeling of now having a body you are happy with!

And then you start to think differently.

"I think I deserve a reward. I think a big bag of chips will do the trick. I'll make up for it tomorrow."

"And why not go for a bit of chocolate later this week? It felt so good to spoil myself a little bit."

"This is fantastic. I'll be able to celebrate my success with my friends this weekend!"

"Now that I think of it, I went a bit overboard with a few meals this week. Hmmm. Oh well, no worries, I'll just exercise more next week."

But, you're convinced you're still following the plan. However, you are starting to gain weight again, day after day, week after week.

"It's not so bad, I only gained two pounds. I'll get back on track next week. Actually, I can't because friends are coming over. The following week then. Oh, but I'm going away on a trip that week. When I get back, for sure. But then the holiday season starts, how could I forget? January it is then. The new year is a great time to get back on track."

Get back on track. There it is. Proof that, thanks to your excuses, you've let everything go. This is how you play yoyo with your weight.

Always be aware of your plan and the behaviours you have to repeat day after day in order to maintain your healthy weight for the rest of your life.

Be aware of the excuses you give yourself. Write them down on a sheet of paper that you can display somewhere you can see it to remind yourself, when you use them, that these are the very same excuses you use to gain weight again.

Losing weight is taking control of your thoughts (and excuses) and your behaviour.

Losing weight is for the hero you have to continue to be... for the rest of your life.

27
STRESS AND EMOTIONS

Yes, life goes on. Sometimes things will go well, and sometimes they won't. Life is such that stress is not completely avoidable. From early childhood to adulthood, you've developed mechanisms to manage stressful situations. Some of these mechanisms are effective, and others not so much.

Eating is a frequently used mechanism to deal with stress and negative emotions. Several of my clients talk to me about their "emotional eating."

The big challenge in this case is to develop a much more effective stress management mechanism. You will have to learn to manage stress otherwise than by binge eating. If you find yourself engaging in "emotional eating," I recommend you see a health care professional (psychologist) who can guide you through this process.

In my opinion, it is very difficult to get over this type of problem on your own. This is why expert help is essential. Since your goal is to maintain your healthy weight for the rest of your life, if you experience this type of problem, you have to resolve it. With no other tools than food to manage stress and emotions, you are at great risk of losing control.

Yes, losing weight forces you to develop better ways of managing stress and emotions.

Losing weight requires personal development work. Losing weight forces you to grow, develop and evolve as a person.

Losing weight is for you, the hero in your own life.

28

YOU WILL OCCASIONALLY FACE INJUSTICE (REAL OR IMAGINED)

How about another discussion with one of my clients to make my point? I see you haven't lost your curiosity!

— Yes, indeed. Your metabolism is slow, among the slowest I've ever measured. But the good news is that you still managed to lose weight since last month: a total of 2 lb.

— Glad you think that's good. I have to limit myself to 1,250 calories a day. I just have to look at a piece of cake and I gain weight.

— *OK... easy does it.* All right, you haven't lost an ounce in the last 4 years, and now that you've lost 2 lb, you're all upset. What am I to understand from that? *But I've already understood everything.*

— My friend eats whatever she wants and she never gains weight. Why should I have to limit myself to 1,250 calories and have to avoid even thinking about a piece of cake?

— *The truth is going to hurt.* Because life is unfair, it's that simple. You have a "micro metabolism" at 900 calories a day, that of a small 160-cm woman who has dieted her entire life. That's reality. Now, you have to decide what to do about it?

— What do you mean?

— Always complaining about your "micro metabolism" won't change anything. You have two choices: follow the plan and get results at the cost of greater sacrifice than another person, or eat whatever you want and live with the weight that will give you.

This is an extreme example, to be sure, but when it comes to weight loss, there is no justice. Complaining about the situation will change nothing. Make a choice and accept living with the consequences.

Here is an example of an "imagined" injustice.

— You know Denis, menopause slows down the metabolism and leads to weight gain.

— *Sometimes, but not always.* Sure, but based on my measurements, your basal metabolism is perfectly normal.

— Then why have I gained 20 lb since I started menopause?

— *Here I go again with the truth.* You're 54 years old. I have a few questions for you. Are your children still living at home?

— No, I live alone with my husband.

— All right then, so now how do you spend all this free time? More romantic meals with plenty of wine perhaps?

— Yes. I must admit that I've developed a real fondness for that glass of wine or two.

— *I really have to ask.* How many drinks do you consume per week?

— Um... only a few glasses, really.

— *I want an exact number.* How many is that?

— I don't want you to think I'm...

— I'm not here to judge you. I'm here to find a solution. So, how many drinks a week?

— My husband and I share a bottle of wine on Thursdays, Fridays and Saturdays, and sometimes on Sundays as well.

— *I'm going to be nice. I won't mention all the sides: appetizers, cheese, dessert.* That is an excellent answer. We finally have a possible solution. According to my estimate, based on your weight, your size, and your metabolism, you shouldn't consume more than 4 glasses of wine per week if you want to lose weight.

— But Denis, I don't know if I feel like reducing the amount of alcohol I drink. Isn't there any other way to lose weight?

— Not to my knowledge.

— That's a bit unfair, what you're asking me to do. Now that I've barely just started to enjoy my free time.

— But I'm not forcing you to do anything. It's up to you to decide. There's nothing unfair about it. It's just reality. You can't just drink and eat as much as you want and lose weight. You know very well that I'm right, and denying the truth won't accomplish anything. It's your decision.

Reaching your healthy weight and maintaining it for the rest of your life means making balanced choices based on the reality imposed by your metabolism. Accepting this reality and acting accordingly is your only possible alternative.

Losing weight is for heroes who can live with the consequences of "their own" reality.

29
YOU HAVE GONE THROUGH A TRANSFORMATION

Imagine a line. At the far left, you have sedentariness and overeating. At the far right, you have food deprivation and high-intensity exercise.

Some people will spend their entire lives at the far left, while others will spin around obsessively at the far right. But at both of these extremes, only imbalance reigns supreme.

**SEDENTARITY
+ OVEREATING**   **FOOD DEPRIVATION +
                                          HIGH-INTENSITY EXERCISE**

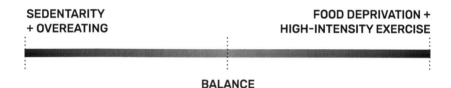

BALANCE

Somewhere in the middle lies your balance ZONE. This balance zone you have found, you'll have to master and maintain throughout the process you have undertaken by reading this book.

In this ZONE, there is nothing very complicated. Oddly enough, this may even sometimes appear too simple a strategy. But as you progress step by step, you will realize that a balanced life is all you really need to achieve your goal.

And, if you look farther ahead, this life strategy you are applying to lose weight can also be applied to every other facet of your life.

As you evolve by reading this book, you will gradually realize that the knowledge and self-mastery you have gained to reach your healthy weight (and maintain it for the rest of your life) can be applied to solve many other problems you will face in your life.

Not only have you lost weight, you have gone through a transformation. You have become a hero.

30
ACCUMULATE SMALL VICTORIES

Some people have become specialists at identifying every detail in their daily lives that confirm that everything is going wrong.

"I hate my body."

"I didn't lose very much weight this month."

"This isn't working."

This type of comment you make every day can only lead to failure and giving up.

Your mental discourse is very important. You want to succeed, so you have to build this success. Focus your attention on the small details that show that you are progressing.

There are two ways to interpret losing one pound (340 grams).

"This is really disappointing, I really expected a lot more."

Or,

"This is great! It's working. I just have to maintain the same strategy and my progress will be steady."

Between these two attitudes, which one do you choose?

Losing weight is for heroes that can savour small victories and accumulate positive results.

31
TEN CHARACTERISTICS
OF PEOPLE WHO SUCCEED

You realize, now, that the end is never the end. Your goal is to achieve a healthy weight and to maintain it for the rest of your life. Over the years, I've advised many people who have achieved this goal. Several years after our first meeting, they still maintain a healthy weight because they continue to apply the behaviours and strategies that led to their success.

All of these people share the same characteristics that you are currently learning to develop:

1. They hold their health and weight loss program as **a top priority**.

2. Like everyone else, they encounter difficulties, but **they persevere**.

3. They give themselves **no excuses** to go back to their old habits. They **tirelessly repeat the behaviours and strategies** that led to their success.

4. They understand that **losing weight is their responsibility** and are not looking for a "miracle method."

5. They understand which **strategies are the most effective** in terms of nutrition and training, based on their metabolism. Deprivation and high-intensity exercise are no longer part of their lifestyle. They have found the proper balance.

6. They have taken the time they needed to understand how their metabolism works and reacts. **They have invested the time they needed to succeed.**

7. They focus their attention on positive results, **as small as they may be**, and not on the appearance of failure.

8. They understand the conditions under which their body loses weight and the conditions under which it gains weight. **They are in control of their weight.**

9. For them, there is no other way to conduct themselves. **They have changed their lifestyle and there is no going back.**

10. Lastly, they have **faced the challenge of "losing weight"** along with everything this requires of them.

These characteristics make you a hero that can succeed and achieve your goal.

Losing weight is for heroes. Losing weight is for you.

32
A HERO'S JOURNEY

Actions speak much louder than words. With regard to weight loss, you now think and act differently. Your actions reveal the person you have become. You will encounter difficulties and experience crises, but they will allow you to reveal your true nature. A solid person who can focus on achieving your objectives. Of course, things will not always be so rosy. You may occasionally stumble, but the important thing is to lift up your head, look straight ahead and get back up.

Losing weight. What started out as the simple notion of shedding a few pounds (or kilos) as quickly as possible has now transformed into a true understanding of what defines change.

In order to reach the real goal (to reach a healthy weight and to maintain it for the rest of your life), you have had to redefine who you are. Losing weight has become an opportunity for you to grow and evolve.

You have seized this opportunity. It has been a long journey. A journey for heroes.

CONGRATULATIONS!

PART 4
YOUR FUTURE

33
HOW TO USE THIS BOOK

You can read this book, and then ignore everything and go back to your old habits, and perhaps tell yourself that the best thing to do might be to look for another "miracle" approach rather than change your lifestyle.

You can read this book, apply the plan as suggested and drop everything in 2 or 3 months.

You can read this book and use it to change your lifestyle and achieve the desired results. Then, a few months or years later, start to gain weight again.

You can read this book and use it to change your lifestyle and achieve your goals. You can also decide to keep it handy, as a constant reminder of the strategies you have to apply on a daily basis to maintain your results... for the rest of your life. For you, there's no going back.

34
CHOOSING YOUR LIFE

You have changed your lifestyle, you have reached your goals and you now know that there are no easy solutions. To maintain your healthy weight, you must tirelessly repeat the same behaviours and pay attention to your nutrition. Lying to yourself is no longer an acceptable solution. You must decide if your new lifestyle is right for you.

What will you be telling yourself in 6 months or a year?

I would like for things to be different ✗	I love my new lifestyle ✓
"It requires a lot of discipline. I can't stay motivated. I don't know if I really feel like living with this type of discipline. I feel like I could enjoy life more. I can no longer eat as much as I want on weekends. I miss that. Life isn't as much fun as it was."	"I love my new lifestyle. I can eat my fill. I've incorporated delicious foods into my nutrition. I am aware of my nutritional choices at all times and I really enjoy feeling in control. I am in control of my weight and I like my body. This is fantastic!"

Remember, you can choose whether or not to follow the plan that led to success, but there is no middle ground. You must choose to eat whatever you want and gain weight or maintain your new lifestyle and stay in control of your weight.

35
YOUR RESULTS IN 3 YEARS

Which of the following statements will represent you in 3 years?

I've gained weight, but it's not that bad	I'm proud of myself
"I've sidetracked from my plan somewhat... Actually, I've gained back all the weight I lost. Maybe more.	"I've been maintaining my healthy weight for three years now. I've really incorporated my new lifestyle.
But, I know that it's not so bad, because now I know what to do to lose weight. I just have to go back to my plan.	I've enjoyed so many benefits to my health, my fitness, my enjoyment of life and my energy that I feel like a totally new person.
I'll go back to my plan when the time is right in my life, however. I'm very busy and I don't really have time to take care of myself right now."	I'm really proud of myself."

36
AND IN 5 YEARS?

Will you still be playing yoyo with your weight or will you still maintain your healthy weight?

It wasn't working for me anymore	I don't even think about it anymore
"I'm sure I was following the plan to the letter, but I've started to gain weight again. It wasn't working for me anymore, so I tried new weight loss methods. What I don't understand, however, is why I manage to lose weight but always gain it back again. There must be something weird with my metabolism."	"I've been following my plan for 5 years now. What fascinates me is how my new lifestyle is so completely incorporated into my daily life that I don't even think about it anymore. Being fit and maintaining a healthy weight has become so simple and natural to me."

37
AND IN 10 YEARS?

Nothing has changed ⊗	Problem solved ⊘
"I've wasted my whole life trying to lose weight."	"I've lost weight once and for all."

38
KEEP THIS BOOK WITH YOU

Yes, you must keep this book with you for the next 10 years. Losing weight is a hero's journey, and even heroes need to remember what led them to success.

Losing weight is a long journey. A journey for heroes.

CONTACT

Dr. Denis Boucher, Ph.D.
www.mycloudbody.com
denis.boucher@mycloudbody.com

26484258R00052

Printed in Great Britain
by Amazon